HAPPINESS

A Little Guide To Self-Love And Positive Thinking

Jill Hesson

TABLE OF CONTENTS

Introduction

Happiness. This is probably the most sought after emotion in the world and yet somehow, despite our abundance of wealth, increase in health and freedom from tyrannical oppression it seems to have grown more elusive. We have confused our quest to find inner peace with our desires for success and financial gain. Again and again the world transmits a message that if you work really hard you will become really successful and from there happiness will be a bi-product that just follows naturally. People in the rich industrialized countries are now wealthier than they have been at any time in our history and yet all the evidence points to the fact that we are now unhappier than we have ever been.

What can it be that we are getting wrong? Why is it that depression levels, even among adolescents, are sky rocketing? We are not the first people to go in search of the answers to this problem. It is an age-old dilemma that dates back thousands of years but which seems to be reaching a crisis level at the moment. The last fifty years have seen huge leaps forward in our knowledge of the workings of the human brain and the psychology associated with it. Science has already answered many of the questions we have in regard to happiness and as you delve deeper into this book you are going to learn that your happiness levels are not just something that happen to you or are the result of the circumstances in which you find yourself. You can develop your brain's receptiveness to happiness in much that same way as you are able to develop your physical stamina: through discipline and effort combined with some education as to how the mind works.

The techniques that you are about to read are not complicated or taxing. They are not dependent on hours of positive reinforcement methodology designed to trick your mind into believing something that it does not want to. In fact, deep down inside, you are about to discover that much of what it takes to be really happy you already knew. It had just become buried beneath a constantly deepening layer of disinformation telling you that happiness equaled money plus success. We are about to bust that myth wide open and offer a different route altogether.

Chapter 1: Busting the More is Better Myth

It is difficult to say where it first started. Perhaps it was with us all along, buried deep in our genes, or perhaps it is just part of our evolutionary makeup that we have carried with us since we first began to walk upright. Where ever it came from, the fact is that human beings the world over seem to believe that effort will lead to wealth and that will in turn inevitably lead to happiness. But what if we have it all wrong? What if wealth and success and all their associated trappings are not the basis of happiness? That would mean that all we have been led to believe, all we have been pursuing in the hunt for happiness might have been in vain. Sure we now have the recognition, the fancy car and the palatial house but are we really happy? All the evidence points to the fact that we are not. Too many rich and famous people are admitting to the fact that they suffer from deep feelings of isolation, emptiness and very often depression. Having clawed their way up the ladder and finally reached what so many of us aspire to they have poked their heads through the clouds and discovered that there is still something missing in their lives. These are the same people that the media is pointing to as demonstrating the pinnacle of success to which we should all aspire.

Most of us live in a fast-moving technological world that puts huge demands on our time. In the early sixties, the impression was that we were on the verge of a mechanical and technological revolution that would see us wondering what to do with all the spare time we suddenly had on our hands. As machines and computers handled many of our daily chores and freed us from the grind and boredom those duties imposed on us, we were expected to suddenly have so much leisure time to deal with that it was feared that boredom would become the overriding issue of the coming decades. Well they sure got that one wrong.

Today our worlds have changed so dramatically that even in our own lifetimes we can see dynamic differences to what we grew up with. Not long ago mobile phones and email were just dreams and now they are so common place they do not even get remarked upon, even in remote third world countries. Their appearance heralded a new era of dynamic communication. No more waiting weeks for a reply to your carefully hand written letter. No more hoping someone was at home to take your call. Now we have instant contact, anytime, anywhere. Eighty percent of us sleep with a mobile phone beside our beds and it is the last thing we check before going to sleep at night.

For those of us old enough to remember the days prior to these now common place innovations we can recall the hopes and aspirations that they produced when they were first trialed. We eagerly looked forward to them but it never even crossed our minds that one day soon we would never be able to escape their clutches. More than ever we are now required to be available twenty-four hours a day, seven days a week. Those moments of peaceful inaccessibility we once enjoyed are now a thing of the past.

I do not wish to lay the blame for our loss of happiness solely at the doorstep of these two means of communication. What I am trying to demonstrate is that somehow our lives have speeded up and we seem to be trying to cram more and more into less and less time and technology and mechanization seem to have added to that pressure. Escape becomes more difficult.

I have just visited a small village in the south of France where I spoke to an old lady who can remember a time when twice a year all the woman of the village would load the washing onto horse drawn carts which were then towed to the communal 'lavoir' or washing area. They would then camp there for two days and do all the washing from the preceding six months and lay it on the grass to dry. I found the comparison fascinating, especially when viewed against our modern lives where every couple of days we toss our dirty clothes into the washing machine before leaping into our cars to start the hour-long commute through the traffic to our cubicle sized offices.

Her washing procedure was so different that I questioned her at length about it. It seemed to me that washing your huge pile of clothes by hand in a stone wash pool fed by a cold stream must have been torturous. What she said really shocked me and drove home to me how much the speed at which we live our modern lives has squeezed out so much happiness. The communal washing was looked forward to, as it was a great communal activity in which the woman all assisted one another but also caught up on each other's news and gossip. To my surprise she looked back on those days with great fondness.

We now have more to wash but at the same time we have developed machinery to make that chore easier, faster and more productive. But what have we lost in comparison to a once much slower pace of life where even doing the household laundry was a communal activity that gave us the opportunity to interact with others. We have bigger houses but mostly they are designed around giving us privacy, which has cut us off from all but the briefest relationship with our neighbors. Our fast-moving high powered cars are all very well but once stuck in the traffic we move at the same mind numbingly slow speed as everyone else.

It is without doubt that as a society we now have more in the way of material goods than at any time in our past history. We also have more than ever in the way of debt and many people are paying a huge psychological price knowing that we have debts to pay at the end of each month. Many of these debts are to pay for goods we often don't need but which were bought in order to give the appearance of wealth to impress friends and neighbors. Shopping has become a sort of short-term therapy. We become depressed through a combination of factors then buy something to relieve the depression. That shiny new purchase gives temporary relief to our woes but the relief soon wears off and we rapidly find the pleasure derived from our new item vanishes. We are then left with more debt to pay and a greater feeling of depression, which triggers the whole cycle again.

The more is better myth also leaves us in no doubt that if we work harder and longer we will eventually rise above all this debt and find ourselves in a position where we have enough not only to clear outstanding bills but an excess that will guarantee us happiness. An interesting statistic comes from winners of large lottery prizes. In a survey of past winners, it was discovered that the majority of them were less happy six months after the draw than they were prior to the big win. Even more interesting was the fact that though they admitted to being less happy none of them would give the prize back.

We learn two important facts from the more is better scenario. One is that those people whose lives we are told to aspire to and who have achieved what the world perceives as success are often not happy. The second is that many people are living their lives on the basis of delayed gratification where instead of being happy now, they labor away at achieving wealth, fame or both on the assumption that happiness will follow. If we want to achieve happiness we must aim at it and not at something else from which we hope happiness will be a bi-product. Happiness must become our primary target not a secondary one and later in this book we will look at ways of accessing that target. First, however we need to take a short look at the brain and how it works.

Chapter 2: How Our Minds Work

If you are going to go after happiness successfully you need to dispel more than just the more is better myth. You need to accept that your attitude toward happiness is not just something you are born with and over which you have no control. If you are stuck in that thought rut you will never be able to change and your happiness will be derived purely from the circumstances that befall you. All of us are constantly being confronted by an ever-changing array of situations and problems and it is how we perceive these that determine whether or not we are to be happy or not. It is often referred to as the glass half full scenario. One person can view an incident and see it as being positive whilst another, when confronted with exactly the same scenario, may perceive it as being negative. We often tend to imagine that this way, in which we perceive things is just part of our makeup and that we cannot adjust that. Science has now proved that this is far from the truth.

The way in which we view situations, in fact, the way that we do anything, is always dictated by our brains. That small organ situated between our ears and which would fit comfortably into the palms of our hands plays a vital part in every activity that our bodies perform. It controls our emotions, our movements and a million other things that very often we are unaware of such as breathing. It is probably the most complex organism in the universe and despite massive leaps forward in our understanding of its functions over the last two decades or so there is still much about it that we simply do not understand.

One thing that we have learned through recent research is that contrary to earlier expectations our brains can change. They can be developed in much the same way as our muscles can be developed and therefore we are not simply stuck with a glass half full, glass half empty mindset. We are the masters of our own mindsets and there is no reason why we should not train our brains to be more receptive toward happiness.

The brain produces one hundred thousand chemical reactions every second. Recent estimates find that we have eighty-six billion cells in this single organ weighing in at less than three pounds and consisting mostly of water. All too often the press comes up with some story of a robot or other form of so called artificial intelligence that they claim is the precursor to a piece of technology that will soon be able to think as clearly as we do. The fact is we are still a million miles away from producing anything technological that has anywhere near the capabilities of performing the tasks that our brains do on a constant day by day basis.

Despite all the wonders our brains have to offer there are still pitfalls that we need to be aware of. Each of us produces an average of fifty thousand thoughts per day. For most people, however, the overriding majority of those thoughts are negative. Researchers have found that we have an almost inbuilt system of negative default to which our brains revert if we do not learn to discipline them. Quite what the reason for this is no one is quite sure. It could be that in order to evolve in a hostile world in which we humans were often seen as prey we naturally had to have thought processes that were cautious and erred toward seeing things in an adverse light. Sheer survival meant that almost everything we encountered had to be viewed with a degree of skepticism.

Regardless of what the reasons are behind this negative thinking default, the fact is that we have to retrain our brains to see things in a more positive light if we are to achieve the levels of happiness that we all hunger for. Much of this is simply down to knowing how the thought processes work and then offering the mind something positive to cling to instead of that negative thought that it naturally errs toward. Our brains are conditioned to only focus on one thing at a time. That is not to say that we can only have one thought at a time. Those of you with wives will no doubt have been assured that women are particularly adept at multi tasking. We are all able to perform tasks on several different levels but most of these tasks are background tasks that can be performed with little attention whilst our brains focus on a single thought. Hence our wonderful ability to walk, talk and chew gum without stopping.

If we are aware that our natural instinct is to throw up a negative thought in the majority of situations and if we know that our brains can only focus on one thought at a time, then it stands to reason that the solution to this problem is within our grasp. We need to replace those negative thoughts with positive ones and that will then fill the space that negative thinking has had free reign in previously. Of course, this is easier said than done but over the course of the next few chapters we will look at some of the primary methods of holding onto sustained positivity that in turn will guide us toward truer happiness. We will start to examine that, but for now the most important thing is that you start to accept that you are able to change the way your brain works. You are able to harness its power to err toward happiness and positive thoughts as opposed to negative thoughts. It is this process of thinking and seeing the world about you that will lead to happiness as opposed to the flawed success, wealth then happiness equation that the world has taken to so readily and with such lack of actual success.

Science has known that reversing the way the brain perceives things is possible for some time now. Research paper after research paper shows that we can learn to be more positive and happier but as with much of new science, it is taking its time for this information to filter down to the man in the street. Scientists are academic by nature and dissemination of their discoveries is often not their strong point. Even so there is a growing awareness in many big companies that we have had the cart before the horse up until now and many of them are beginning to focus on employee happiness as a means to greater happiness, creativity and productivity. In short they have begun to reverse that flawed equation we have been using for far too long. Fast growing and out of the box companies like Google, Amazon and Facebook are breaking the mold in terms of how they treat their staff. Hours are more flexible, dress codes have gone out the window, employees are encouraged to bring pets to work and sport and massages are now all part of their new company culture. The results have been overwhelmingly positive. Now it is time for you to start doing the same thing.

Chapter 3: Follow Your Thoughts

As we have seen in the previous chapter, this wonderful tool we have called the brain is capable of doing the most amazing things. Despite all that it is capable of though, we need to be aware of its naturally occurring default setting toward the negative. This will vary between different people and under differing circumstances so that even the most positive thinker will have days where he becomes trapped by negative thought processes that can derail his or her quest for happiness.

Once we are aware that this negative thinking will take place we need to take action to control that. First of all, we need to get into the habit of following our own thought processes so that we can see where they are taking us and discover if there are patterns when we are more vulnerable to off course thoughts. Some of us are more prone to thinking negatively at night or have negative thoughts triggered more easily when driving in heavy traffic for example. A very common time to find yourself drowning in negative thinking is at night when a problem you may be having wakes you or prevents you getting to sleep in the first place.

If you are unaware that this is a natural process it can be very isolating as you feel yourself becoming submerged by your darkest thoughts and do not realize that we are all prone to poor thinking habits from time to time. As your ability to recognize not only where these thoughts are going but also when they are most likely to affect you so you are better equipped to counteract them. When you find yourself becoming more experienced at dealing with these thoughts you will learn to start working backwards from the negative thought to its source and by retracing your mental footprints you are able to return to the last positive thought and start again on a more managed route.

Part of the negative thinking process is what is known as catastrophizing. In this situation, we take a scenario and then imagine the worst possible conclusion. For example, were we to be preparing to give a talk in front of a large and unfamiliar audience we might start to imagine all the worst possible things that could happen. These thoughts become self-perpetuating if not managed correctly. Because of the nervousness generated by our thoughts we subsequently deliver the talk badly and thus come to see ourselves as poor public speakers.

Once we understand that every action we take is governed by our brains and we are only able to hold onto one thought at a time, we can start to feed ourselves with positive self-affirming images. In the same way that the negative thoughts may have led to a disastrous presentation, the positive thoughts could conversely lead to a very successful one as the speaker comes across as happy and self assured. These positive images need not be simply images of ourselves succeeding in adverse situations. Tests have shown that any happy thoughts we are able to conjure up will improve our ability to perform. In other words, the nervous would-be speaker could improve his chances of performing well by imagining himself standing in front of his audience and giving a superb speech. He could have equally successful results if he were to read some amusing anecdotes or mentally transport himself to a place that he finds beautiful and relaxing in the run up to the talk.

The University of Toronto ran numerous tests in respect to emotions affecting behavior. They have concluded that happiness leads to increases in both serotonin and dopamine to the brain. This in turn activates the learning centers in the brain resulting in better creativity and thinking processes.

In a series of tests among four year olds, one group was encouraged to conjure up positive and happy images before performing a task whilst another was not primed at all. The primed group significantly outperformed the non-primed group. Similar tests were delivered to a wide variety of other groups including students and adults and in all cases those primed with positive thoughts performed better. Other tests show that happy thoughts even improve our vision. In experiments, again conducted by the University of Toronto, the subjects who were positively primed were more observant of images and showed greater visual cortex activity than those who were not primed.

To put this into its most simple terms our negative thoughts are related to our ancient fight or flight reaction. We are preprogrammed to imagine the worst-case scenario so that we can rapidly defend ourselves or flee according to the circumstances. Imagination is one of those areas where we differ from other animals. It is what makes us creative and leads us to be inventive and logical. It can also work against us if we allow our imaginings to be dominated by negative scenarios. Instead we need to have a catalogue of positive thoughts and images we can project onto our minds each time we follow it and find it leading us in a negative direction. Simply trying to extinguish the negative thought will not work. Our brains cannot deal with a vacuum and negative images need to be replaced by positive ones.

At first this will be a little difficult. Even as you start to develop your armory of positive images your mind will be trying to tell you that this project will not work and that you should give up. With a bit of practice, you will find that you become better at detecting the negative thoughts and replacing them with positive ones. The better you become the less negative thoughts you will have as your mind starts to drop into the new habit of seeing the positive more quickly. You will also begin to realize how many of the negative thoughts that you had conjured up over the years never actually occurred. Suddenly you are on the road to finding a happy you and you didn't even have to buy a new car to get there.

Chapter 4: Try a Little Gratitude

Scientists have made the rather unexpected discovery that grateful people tend to worry less and live longer. Most of us tend to look around and notice all the things we do not have. We see one of the neighbors has just bought a new car on the one side of us; another has put on an extension to his house on the other side whilst the one across the road has just had a whole range of new appliances delivered. We immediately look at our own unchanged circumstances and imagine that we are being deprived in some way.

In our careers, we tend to do the similar thing. We look at the person one or two rungs further up the corporate ladder than we are and we envy them. It has been revealed that whilst we may dream of being the next rock star, sporting hero or billionaire, it is not these larger than life characters that most affect our self esteem. Whilst we may have aspirations of massive success in general we accept its un-attainability. The person we most want to impress is the guy next door or in the next office. These are targets we see as attainable and it is where we direct most of our gaze and most of our envy if they outperform us in some way.

An important thing to come to terms with when searching for happiness is that no matter how high up the ladder we climb or how much we accumulate there will always be someone a little higher than us or a little wealthier than us. To constantly envy those people is a recipe for unhappiness, poor relationships and consuming jealousy. There is a Taoist saying that states 'he who knows he has enough is rich.' Most members of the human race however are insatiable. In contrast to the Taoist saying take a look at this statement by

John D. Rockefeller when asked how much is enough? 'Just a little bit more.' At the time, he was considered to be the richest person in modern history.

I doubt any of us are ever going to be able to compete with Rockefeller in terms of wealth but there is absolutely no reason not to be as happy as or happier than he was despite his massive wealth. We need to change the way we look at things. I suspect that one or two readers are shaking their heads and saying that I have no idea how tough their lives actually are. Well, I have no desire to demean or diminish the desperate situation that some may find themselves in but let's just take a brief moment to look at some of the things we do have to be grateful for right now.

Twenty six percent of the world is illiterate and would not be able to read this book or any other for that matter.

One in nine people do not have enough food to lead healthy active lives.

783 million people do not have access to clean water.

2.5 billion do not have adequate sanitation.

There are 100 million homeless people and that figure rises to 1000 million who are in temporary or insecure housing.

Who cares what car the neighbor is driving? If we are to achieve happiness we need to start to see things with different eyes. We need to start to look down the ladder instead of up it and we must stop seeing what we do not have and start to be more grateful for all that we do have. By sheer nature of the birth lottery we have been born with so much more than the vast majority of the people on this planet.

Gratitude is good for us and is something we do not even need to take in large doses. Try to start off each morning by thinking of three things to be grateful for before you even get out of bed in the morning. They do not need to be big things or earth shattering discoveries. Perhaps you just had a good night's sleep after a series of restless nights. Perhaps you can hear the patter of little feet from the room next door as a child gets ready for school. This is not something that someone else can really show you. You need to find your own sources of gratitude but you also need to train yourself to search them out.

Once you have got out of bed try to remind yourself to look for little triggers of gratitude during the course of your day. It does not really matter how large or small these things are. The issue here is that you are reprogramming that mind of yours to look for them. This will not only provide you with small moments of happiness throughout the course of the day but it also performs the vitally important task of dragging your mind away from its favorite negative default setting. Filling your mind with gratefulness leaves no room for negative thoughts to gain a toehold.

Chapter 5: Kindness Counts

One unexpected source of happiness comes from doing things for others. It sounds counter intuitive that in searching for happiness of our own we can get closer to our goals by performing small acts of random kindness toward other people. Researchers have found that even seemingly minor acts of kindness can reap rewards out of proportion to the acts themselves when it comes to achieving happiness.

Try looking for an opportunity to do something kind or generous at least once per day. It need not be an act that is recognized by the recipient but it should be something that you do deliberately. It is not the gratitude of the recipient that generates the feeling of happiness, it is the knowledge that you have chosen to do something for someone else that you might not otherwise have done.

I knew a man who would wear his watch on his right wrist until he had performed an act of kindness each day. He told me that as it was his habit to look at the time by looking at his left wrist he would frequently be reminded if he had not completed his self-imposed assignment and as soon as he had done so he would transfer the watch back to its more familiar position on his left wrist. After a few weeks, he became confident that looking to perform good deeds had become an ingrained habit and he was no longer obliged to use the aide de memoir.

That in many ways is the point. By training our minds through repetition, they quickly adapt to a new circumstance and in this case the newly learned habit provides the reward of a happier mindset. You will make another interesting discovery after several weeks of practicing this discipline; performing acts of kindness will start to become second nature so that you will find yourself automatically looking for opportunities to be kind throughout the day and not just in an attempt to gain self-reward.

The benefits of being kind are not just limited to hearsay evidence. Researchers at the University of British Columbia have shown that by performing acts of kindness there was a significant increase in the positive mood of the person performing the act. Doctor Richard R. Hamilton has demonstrated that an act of kindness releases a hormone known as oxytocin, which generates a feeling of warmth in the brain.

So even if it is just helping an elderly person carry their shopping bags across the car park or helping your child with their homework, always be aware of the fact that these little acts are opportunities to benefit yourself. It provides interesting food for thought when we imagine what a different place our world might be if more people were aware of this potential happiness benefit they could be getting. Simple acts of kindness have an extra benefit in that they are infectious and people who have benefitted from kindness tend to be kinder toward others.

Chapter 6: Meditation

Meditation is an often misinterpreted practice that has been promoted by most of the major religions of the world. I am not advocating that you go off to Asia and spend months in an ashram under the close supervision of some self-proclaimed guru. What I am suggesting is five to ten minutes of each day being spent in quiet stillness to allow your batteries to recharge, as it were. Simply being still and quiet is something we do very seldom in the hustle and bustle of our modern lives.

Instead many of us tend to wake up each morning and then hit the floor running. Many people leap out of bed, rush through their ablutions then gulp down their breakfast before driving through the wall to wall traffic and following that with intense days at the office or whatever work place it is at which they make their income. Most people do not need to be told that somehow this is not conducive to the state of their happiness. They know this instinctively and yet somehow they continue in this vicious cycle, knowing deep down that what they are doing is probably not good for them. Given a bit more time to themselves they might eventually work out some way to extricate themselves from their predicament but time seems to be the one commodity nobody has these days. Even our moments of so called relaxation are normally accompanied by the constant white noise of the television or social media intrusions, or both.

Ten minutes per day of simply sitting quietly focusing on nothing other than breathing slowly in and out has been proven to have dramatic and positive effects on our physical and mental health. There are thousands of books out there dedicated to nothing other than how to meditate but becoming a world-class meditator is not the objective of this book so I will keep it simple. Get up ten minutes earlier than you would normally do and find yourself a comfortable place to sit where you will not be disturbed. Once you are comfortable close your eyes and try to think of nothing. Breathe slowly and deeply. Because you are not accustomed to doing this it will seem like the hardest thing in the world at first.

Your mind will immediately throw distractions at you. And you will find yourself planning the rest of the day or worrying about something that happened at the office the day before. Don't be surprised at this. Your mind is not accustomed to being given a little time off and it is unsure what to do with the sudden gap that has appeared suddenly in its overcrowded schedule. Keep you breathing fairly deep and steady and keep dragging your mind back to that deep breathing process. Follow each breath closely so that you can feel the air moving through your sinuses down into your lungs and abdomen.

For the first few days it is likely that you will find simply sitting still and letting go of your thoughts is very difficult. Some people find that it helps to have a pen and paper handy so that each time the mind reminds them of something they ought to be doing they can write it down and then let go of it until after the meditation session. Having thoughts that bounce from one thing to another is to be expected during the first few days and weeks as you develop the skill of meditating and work out systems that work best for you personally. Just as with any other skill you will improve as long as you practice regularly and persist.

The benefits of meditation are so great that it is no wonder that so many books and videos have been produced on the subject. There has also been a huge amount of scientific research put into its study. MRI scans on people doing meditation shows an increase in areas controlling metabolism and studies on Buddhist monks after long term meditation show that there have been lasting changes to the brain particularly in those areas involving attention, memory and conscious perception.

Meditation can lower blood pressure and heart rate, as well as relieve stress and pain. There has been a lot of interest from education experts recently particularly in schools where there have been discipline and behavioral problems. Some of them have introduced two sessions of meditation into the daily syllabus and they are reporting positive results in regards to both attendance and concentration levels.

The evidence points so powerfully toward the positive benefits of meditation that it has been integrated into the schedules of such companies as Apple, Google and Anderson Cooper.

There are many different techniques and methods and you will need to research which work best for you but I highly recommend incorporating at least ten minutes of meditation somewhere into your daily routine.

Chapter 7: Relationships

Loneliness cannot only damage your attempts to find happiness, it can kill you. Researchers at Brigham Young University have found that low levels of social interaction are the equivalent to smoking fifteen cigarettes per day, not exercising or being an alcoholic. It increases your health risks by twice as much as obesity does. This research is indicative of the whole spectrum of age groups and is not restricted to the elderly. In sharp contrast, research amongst communities with the longest life spans now seems to indicate that it has less to do with diet or air quality than is does with social interaction. Those people who attain a ripe old age do so because they are surrounded by caring communities. The old adage that no man is an island applies very aptly to our happiness. It is much harder to be happy if you do not have some sort of group with whom you can share and on whom you can lean in times of need. We all need support from time to time and if we are integrated into some sort of community then that support group should exist.

Not everyone is blessed with a happy family or large group of friends. We may have lost loved ones because of a death or through some other reason and suddenly find ourselves isolated. In order to achieve happiness, it is going to be important to re-establish or rebuild some sort of group with whom you can develop and inter-relate. For some people this may be very hard to do. When you are alone it becomes easier to become depressed and to cocoon yourself in your own little world. Very few people have the ability to find happiness in these circumstances and it is crucial to re-establish some sort of meaningful contact with a group with whom you can interact. Doing this may take some effort on the part of the person who suddenly finds him or herself alone, but never the less it needs to be done.

Whether you join a church or a sports club, take art classes or dance lessons it is crucial that you do something that is proactive. It may be uncomfortable at first but you will soon find that you become more at ease once you get to know a few people. The most common thing among depressed people is to retreat into their shells and cut themselves off from others but this absolutely the wrong thing to do. No matter how uncomfortable it may be, you must get out there and interact with other people. Social media has made it easier than ever to find groups with whom you can find a common interest. There seems to be no end to the number of forums and communities to which you can attach yourself. As useful as these sites are, make sure that you use them as stepping stones toward more real intercommunity relationships and don't just use them as a replacement. They serve their purpose but they are not a substitute for genuine community interaction.

Social relationships can lead to a fifty percent increase in your chances of longevity. They are a shared benefit in that in gaining happiness through interaction with others we also provide them with the benefit of being able to relate to us and this feeds into the same sort of two-way reward system that I mentioned in the chapter on kindness. Our interactions with others give us the sense of belonging to a larger community and that in turn increases our sense of purpose and overall well-being.

Most researchers and scientists now agree that relationships are crucial to our overall well-being and therefore to our level of happiness. If you are sincere in your desire to increase your levels of happiness, then it might be time to consider expanding your social connections no matter how uncomfortable this may be in the beginning.

Chapter 8: Exercise

The purpose of this book is not to help you gain three pounds of muscle in just eight weeks or lose eight pounds of fat in just three weeks. This is not a book that focuses on physical fitness other than where it overlaps with happiness and it does that on a number of levels. Moderate levels of exercise actually increase our energy levels, stimulate our minds and give us a sense of achievement and well-being. Group exercise is great way to expose ourselves to some of the other community benefits that we looked at in the previous chapter.

Exercise increases the mood enhancing endorphins reaching our brains and studies at the University of Vermont indicate that twenty minutes of exercise see positive results that continue for up to twelve hours. In addition to the well-known physical benefits that we gain through exercise there are significant benefits to our mental health. According to the US Department of Health and Human Services even a short walk can improve our moods whilst thirty to sixty minutes of exercise taken between three and five times per week can have a pronounced effect on our mental health.

A single thirty-minute exercise session is better for your morale than three ten minute sessions. Exercise taken out doors provides more advantages still. It allows us to interact with nature more closely and exposes us to unfiltered sunlight, which can also boost levels of happiness.

So profound are the effects of exercise on our mental well being that the University of Carolina calculates that up to nineteen percent of divorces could have been avoided if both partners had exercised regularly.

It is not necessary to engage in exhausting or physically demanding tasks and if you are new to exercise in general then it may be best to avoid these altogether or at least until you feel ready to up your effort level. Instead aim for a steady paced moderate form of exercise that gets you breathing fast but not panting. I break my exercise regime into two distinct categories: hard physical exercise such as mountain biking or jogging, which is aimed purely at increasing my physical fitness and endurance, and more moderate exercise, which I use to relax and collect my thoughts. Personally, I find nothing beats walking in this regard and even when I am travelling for business purposes I try to incorporate walks of at least half an hour at a time into my schedule. I am prepared to forgo the harder physical exercise but the moderate exercise for my state of mind is just too important to skip. So ingrained has walking become in my lifestyle that I feel stodgy and drowsy if I do not get my daily half hour fix.

Researchers have proved that exercise increase your enthusiasm and feelings of excitement and I am convinced that after even just a few weeks of forcing yourself to take walks every day or two you will find that the routine becomes one that you look forward to. If you really have trouble keeping up the motivation levels, then think about getting a dog. They are great companions and they are relentless and unforgiving in their ability to get you walking. You will also find they are great icebreakers in respect to meeting other people. Strangers will happily come and talk to you if you are accompanied by a cute and friendly looking dog. (Actually they might not talk to you but they will talk to your dog and this affords you the opportunity to talk to them.)

If the mere thought of walking leaves you cold, then look at the vast range of other options that are available to you. I choose walking for its convenience, because it exposes me to nature and because it allows my mind free range to wander where it wants to. I don't need special equipment or need to pay expensive membership fees and I am not tied to any particular arena or area in which to participate in my chosen sport. Though walking in a natural setting is my preferred option I can just as easily walk in a city. I can't even think of many places where it is not possible to get some walking in. You may prefer the gym environment or salsa classes where you are virtually guaranteed to increase your social contacts. What sport you choose is not important. Don't be coerced in any particular direction but instead choose something that you want to do. Any form of exercise is going to demand a level of self-discipline, especially in the beginning, and this will be so much easier if you are engaged in an activity that you enjoy. The main issue here is that you take on board just how crucial a part exercise plays in your overall pursuit of increased happiness.

Chapter 9: Some Extra Suggestions

Sleep

It can be hard to raise your level of happiness if you are not getting sufficient sleep. This is also a bit of a chicken and egg problem because it can be difficult to get enough sleep if you are unhappy. Lying in bed tossing and turning whilst fretting over a problem can leave you feeling more tired and depressed than if you just get up and do something so if you are not sleeping then try sitting up in bed and reading for half an hour. Meditating for five minutes before going to sleep is another excellent technique.

Live in the moment

Many of our worries stem from our ability to imagine the worst-case scenario. Sometimes we need to let go of things. Start to train yourself to release memories from the past that you cannot possibly change and to stop anticipating all the disastrous possibilities that could befall you in the future. Remember your mind cannot hold onto more than one thing at a time so focus on the here and now and find a few immediate reasons to be grateful.

Simply say no

Some people have a gift for dumping their problems in other people's laps. Others have a weakness for taking on every task that they are asked too. Carrying someone else's problems or committing yourself to jobs that were not really yours in the first place are sure fire tracks to lowering your happiness level. You need to learn to recognize the sort of people that are most likely to do this to you but more importantly you need to develop the ability to simply say no. There is no need to be rude or aggressive about this, nor do you need to get caught up on a guilt trip. A simple but polite no will suffice. If the task they are asking you to perform is one that they should be performing themselves or if it should be placed in the hands of someone else, then there is no need to explain your refusal. Decline politely and then leave them with the job of justifying why they should burden you with a job that is not yours in the first place.

Lean toward forgiveness

Forgiving is a great talent to cultivate, if for no other reason than when you carry a grudge it is you that does the carrying and not the person at whom you aim your anger. Grudge carrying grinds away at our souls like a piece of grit in an engine and I have seen many people poison their own lives through their inability to just let go of something. In many instances the grievance may be totally justified, but that inability to let go of it is harming you and may not be bothering the offending party in the least. If that is the case take a few minutes to examine the root cause, turn it over in your mind then make a conscious decision to let go of it and don't go there again. When it pops up its head again, as it will from time to time, just push it out of your mind and focus on more positive thoughts.

Another area of forgiveness that we need to work on is forgiving ourselves. We have all made wrong turns during our lives. We have done things we are ashamed of, have made stupid mistakes or said things that we should not have done. Guilt is not a domain exclusive to you. Sometimes we get the opportunity to put these things right but very often we don't. Be a little bit kind to yourself. Nobody is perfect and perhaps it is time to show yourself a bit of self-loving and simply turn the page. Often these wounds that we carry are the hardest to let go of and if there is no way that you are able to overcome this problem on your own then find someone that you really trust and talk through the problem with them. It is amazing how cathartic talk can be and if the person you open up to is wise and sympathetic they may be able to shine a new light on the problem so that you are able to see it from a different angle.

Connect with nature

In many ways, man has done an amazing job of molding his environment to suit his needs. Even at our very best though, nothing we have managed to construct can compete with the beauty and sheer grandeur of nature. Exposing yourself to wild empty spaces is a tonic to our moods. Sitting watching the sunset over the sea, listening to birds calling or walking through the forest and noticing the wild flowers can do more to boost morale than we imagine sometimes. The great bounty of offerings provided by nature is often free and just needs to be utilized. To fully take advantage of this bounty, however, we need to train ourselves to see with all our senses. Just as the great wine connoisseurs can take a small sip of wine and then list all its qualities, so too we must learn to extract all that the pallet of nature provides us.

Don't just trudge through the woods as though it is a chore to complete as quickly and efficiently as possible. Look out for small flowers or mushrooms, listen for bird calls and notice the smell of damp leaves that mold away on the forest floor and bring new life in the process. Happiness is an appreciation of an amalgamation of small details rather than just big moments.

Learn to fail

Lose your fear of failure. It is holding you back from a full life. Stop taking on only the things at which you know you will succeed. Life is an adventure and if you see it as such it opens up so many opportunities. We all have a desire to do well at the tasks that lie before us but there is a limit to the things we are going to be good at. Sometime life is just too short to only do what you know will turn out well. Take those piano lessons, write that book or learn a new language. We regret the things we have not done more than the things we have done. Don't find yourself on your deaths bed saying I wish I had tried that. Understand that society is a conservative master. It will always try to force you down the paths most travelled and exaggerate the benefits of doing what everyone else does. Do not cower to social rules. Write your own.

Live in the present

Too many people are living sad unfulfilled lives on the assumption that at some stage down the road they will have the time or money to find the happiness that they know they are missing out on now. How terribly sad. I have bad news for those people. They are going to die. I know that I am too but I don't want to die waiting to live. Seize every opportunity to live while you can and you are sure to be happier overall than you will be if you hope to bank that happiness for a later date. That would be a workable solution if you knew the exact time that you were going to die but most of us don't know that. Those that do, normally due to the onset of a terminal illness of some kind, tend to offer the same advice; live while you can, appreciate the small things in life and spend time with those you love. You seldom hear of anyone with a fatal disease suggesting to others that they should work really hard, build up a good pension fund and find a nice retirement home to die in.

Simplify everything

In a million different ways, we have become accustomed to over complicating our lives. We buy homes that are bigger than what we need then spend hours cleaning them, maintaining them or fretting because we don't have the time we need to do either. In the process, we take on a huge debt that we will often be tied to for the remainder of our lives. In doing so we depriving ourselves of the freedom to stop work when we want to or forcing us to continue in jobs that give us nothing other than a pay check to service the debt for the overly large house.

We fill that house with stuff, which we don't use or need and that adds to our debts and our depression. In order to alleviate the depression, we go out and buy a flash new car that will impress the neighbors. It provides light relief for a few weeks but the novelty soon wears off we are left paying for it for the next five years. Our neighbors are not too impressed because they understand how much we have gone into debt to get that car. They, after all, tried the same trick on you last year so they know exactly where this is coming from. Pretty soon the whole neighborhood is in debt up their eyeballs and nobody is really happy.

Your scenario may not have played out in exactly this fashion but look around you. Consumerism is not only robbing us of happiness and it is destroying the environment and creating broken societies. Train yourself to want less and you will have taken a massive step toward a happier life.

Learn to love yourself

We all carry emotional baggage. Old hurts and scars that we hide from the outside world but which are still there. Some of these wounds stem from those who have hurt us but often they stem from feelings derived from things that we may have done or failed to do. We need to be honest with ourselves and examine just how much these wounds are effecting our attempts at happiness. For most of us the answer is going to be not very much, but there are some who will be suffering on an ongoing basis. Those people need to learn to let go of this and recognize that nobody is perfect and you cannot change the past. Start feeding your mind with positive images about yourself and focus on the good things you have done, are doing and plan to do. Only by fully converting to a positive mindset and letting go of self-blame will you be able to move forward. You need to remember that not just in order to increase your access to personal happiness, but also because in failing to live up to being the best person you can be you may be depriving those around you from seeing you flourish.

Listen to your inner voice

If you are someone doing something you know you ought not to be doing, then your happiness is at stake. From time to time everyone moves outside of their personal moral boundaries and hopefully they correct their course and carry on in a way that is more comfortable to their consciences. Others however pursue activities that they know goes against what they believe in but for one reason or another they continue with that self-destructive behavior. Think of those with gambling or alcohol addictions or who are caught up in extra marital affairs for example. Some people can live their lives in these conditions but that is rare. Most of us become troubled by a guilty conscience. We can continue the behavior but there will always be that small inner voice that disrupts our access to total happiness. In these cases, we need to cease the behavior even if it requires professional help otherwise real happiness will always prove elusive.

Conclusion

Despite its hunger for material goods, happiness is the Holy Grail that society is really searching for. Aiming at wealth and assuming that you will find happiness is like shooting at one target and hoping to hit the bull's eye on another. It simply does not make sense. The media has played a pivotal role here by offering so many glitzy celebrities as role models to aspire to, despite the fact that most of them show little sign of having achieved true happiness. The sad thing is that I do not think the media is trying to create a sort of propaganda message when it does this. Instead I fear that it actually believes in the misguided message that it delivers so widely.

What this book has set out to show is that happiness is achievable without vast quantities of fame or fortune. It lies just at our fingertips waiting to be seized, but we need to re-educate our minds in order to fully enjoy it. Happiness is not dependent on the size of our bank accounts or the type of car we drive. Instead we need to learn to see the value of the little everyday pleasures that surround us. We need to value community, let go of our fears and negative thought processes and practice kindness toward others. As children, we had these abilities but somewhere in the process of becoming adults we have bought into a myth that was never really true in the first place.

None of the exercises and methods in this book are overly demanding, expensive or difficult. They require you to pay attention to your thought processes, give yourself a few minutes each day to simply be quiet and still and take a walk in the woods from time to time. Happiness is largely subjective and each of us chooses to see the glass as being half full or half empty. There is a certain amount of retraining of the mind and discipline required but the reward is that you will be able to live and laugh more freely. If you do choose to follow the advice in this book you hold the keys to happiness in the palm of your hands. Be careful how you use it; it can infect others!

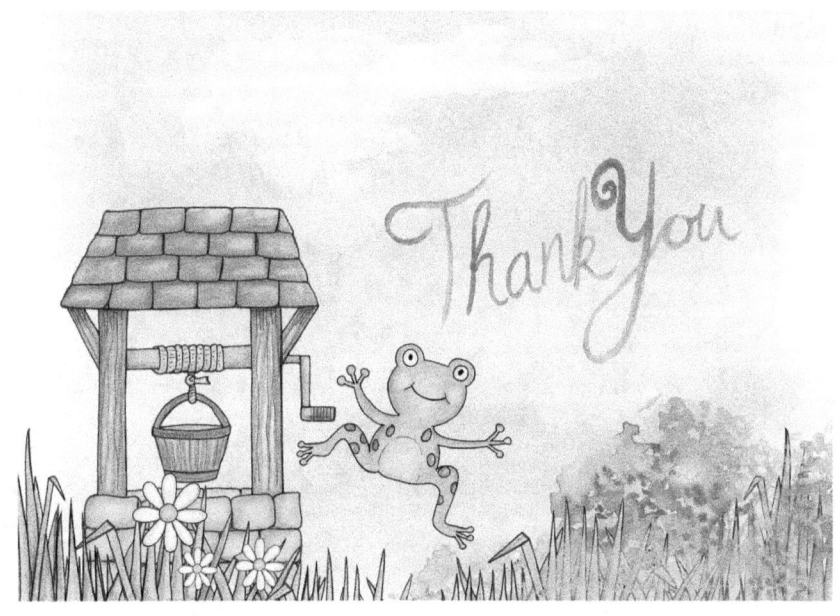

Finally, if you enjoyed this book, then I'd like to ask you for a favor, would you be kind enough to leave a review for this book on Amazon? It'd be greatly appreciated!

Click here to leave a review for this book on Amazon!

https://goo.gl/gl1uW0

Thank you and good luck!

Preview Of

'Yoga: 4-Week Step By Step Guide for Yoga Beginners'

Introduction

We live in a world where we feel completely lost and just riding along. We feel as if we just exist without any particular purpose in life. When that happens, anxiousness, stress and depression starts creeping in, and we stop taking care of how we look as well as our health. The result is an unhealthy lifestyle, which may even advance to various health complications. Have you gotten to that point of your life where you feel you need to find your purpose and bring order to your currently disorderly life?

Well, yoga can do all that since it can help you to bring the much needed order in your physical, mental and spiritual life. What do you think yoga is? Do you think of it as simply executing Olympics level gymnastics stunts? Well, yoga is much more than these stunts. This book will introduce you to yoga, what it is all about and how you can start practicing yoga in as little as 4 weeks.

The Basics

"*Yoga*" is a Sanskrit word formed from a Latin word '*yoke*' meaning to join. From a human perspective, the easiest way to understand yoga is to view it as a union of various aspects of the human spirit and body such as the physical, mental, and spiritual being.

In simpler language, we can define yoga as spiritual techniques and exercises that are designed to 'join' your body and mind. It also can help you attain oneness with the universe. Yoga also helps you achieve a healthier lifestyle because it facilitates weight loss, improves blood circulation, and boosts your flexibility.

As we shall see later in the book, different yoga techniques and Asanas demand for specific approaches to derive the expected benefits: unification of various aspects of the human spirit.

In this guide, we shall look at yoga from a varied perspective in a bid to help you derive the benefits offered by yoga.

Before we start discussing how to practice yoga, let us look at the benefits you stand to gain by practicing yoga. By looking at these benefits, you will feel inspired to start your 4-week Yoga challenge.

Why Practice Yoga?

Yoga uses various spiritual and physical exercises that bring many benefits to yoga yogis and yoginis (these are the respective names given to male and female yoga practitioners). For instance, yoga is useful for weight loss, building muscles, relieving stress, and strengthening the heart.

Regular practice can also help you achieve inner peace especially if you pair yoga with meditation. If you are looking for a refreshing leisure activity, yoga can still be an interesting exercise you can practice alone or with friends. Whatever reason you may have for wanting to become a yogi or yogini, yoga can deeply connect your mind, body, and spirit, which can help you experience your real self.

Let us detailedly discuss the various benefits yoga has for its practitioners:

1. Boosts Physical Fitness

Yoga uses various poses and stretches; what we call asanas. Research shows that holding asanas for at least 60 seconds can boost your posture and deadlift strength. Yoga can boost balance of strength onto your opposing muscle groups, and help you improve flexibility and range of motion.

The good thing is that yoga poses are simple and can fit everyone ranging from body builders, athletes, the obese, and members of either gender. When practiced properly, yoga reduces stress buildup in the muscles, relaxes you, and prevents possible workout injuries because it improves flexibility.

To benefit from yoga in terms of strength gains, elongated muscles, and boosting physical fitness, its best to adopt yoga as part of your regular workout program. For instance, doing yoga stretches before strength training allows the muscles to freely workout without actually shutting down in response to stretched tendons.

Better still, yoga aids movement through your full range of motion when hitting weights. With a full range of motion, you can build long and full-toned muscles or abs. Physical fitness experts are of the view that stretching yoga poses elongate the protective heath of connective tissues that cover muscles and its cells and repair worn out muscles.

The main reason why yoga energizes and strengthens muscle groups is the long deep breaths, something you have to do as you practice yoga asanas. These deep breaths supply oxygen to the muscles, and boost your ability to focus on workouts.

Yoga can fit into a busy or sedentary lifestyle. Further, some research shows that yoga can heal chronic pain such as migraines. Without much effort, a beginner yogi such as yourself can learn how to make informed health choices and practice specific yoga asanas and techniques aimed at improving your health. This lifestyle coaching can include various aspects like stress reduction, exercising, diet, mindfulness, and other relaxation techniques.

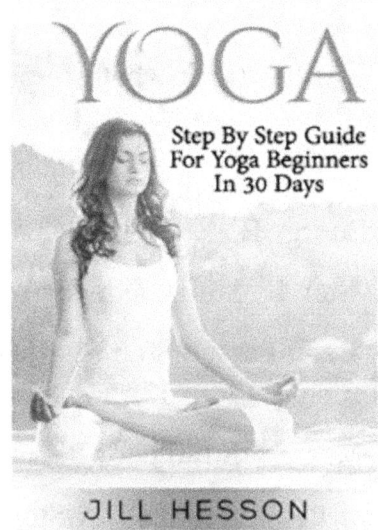

http://amzn.to/2bBlfTw

Here Is A Preview Of What You Can Learn From This Book.

- The Basics of Yoga
- Why Practice Yoga?
- How to Adopt Yoga in 4 weeks: A Three Step Approach
- 4-Week Step By Step Guide

Check out the rest of the book by searching for this title on Amazon website.

Check Out My Other Books

Below you'll find my other books that are popular on Amazon and Kindle as well.

- Chakras For Beginners: The 7 Chakras Guide On How to Balance your Energy Body through Chakra Healing

- Yoga: 4-Week Step By Step Guide for Yoga Beginners

- Buddhism for Beginners: 8 Step Guide to Finding Peace and Enlightenment in Your Life

- Ultimate Self-Mastery Bundle for Beginners 3 in 1 Bundle

- Mindfulness for Beginners: 21-Day Step By Step Guide to Relieve Stress and Find Peace in Your Everyday Life

- Happiness: A Little Guide To Self-Love And Positive Thinking

www.ingramcontent.com/pod-product-compliance
Lightning Source LLC
Chambersburg PA
CBHW070232290526
45789CB00004B/1598